29 Weeks

E. F. C. Warden

ISBN: 1535389117
ISBN-13: 978-1535389112

DEDICATION

For Remi and Daniel -
both of whom teach me patience on a daily basis.

TABLE OF CONTENTS

Acknowledgments   i

1   Introduction   1

2   29 Weeks   2

3   30 Weeks   14

4   31 Weeks   18

5   32 Weeks   23

6   33 Weeks   30

7   34 Weeks   33

8   35 Weeks   39

9   36 Weeks   46

10   37 Weeks   58

11   38 Weeks   61

12   39 Weeks   63

13   Birth   65

14   Postpartum   67

ACKNOWLEDGMENTS

I would like to thank my husband, Daniel, who listened to
me whine and answered all my annoying, repetitive
questions. I would, also, like to thank all of my family and
friends who have supported me over the years

*"God grant me the serenity
to accept the things I cannot change;
courage to change the things I can;
and wisdom to know the difference."*

Reinhold Niebuhr

!

1: INTRODUCTION

At 29 weeks pregnant I was diagnosed with preterm labor and hospitalized for a week. The doctor was able to stop my labor and sent me home on medicine and bed rest. Throughout this period of time I decided to document my bed rest by writing letters to my unborn daughter; letters to help me cope with everything happening.

These are those letters.

2: 29 WEEKS

Dear Remi,

Hello. This is the first official letter I'll ever write to you. So, please allow me to write a formal greeting. Hello little girl, I am your mother. One day we will meet and you will know me the way I hope to one day know you, but for now allow these letters to be what ties us here in this moment and opens a window between us while we wait for that day when you arrive here safe and sound.

First off I wanted to tell you about my day. Currently I'm lying in a hospital bed where I am tethered by multiple machines placed here to keep you safe. I've been here for nearly three days and may not be leaving any time soon. But don't fret little dove, all is well and they tell me it may only be another day before you, daddy, and I can go home. I will most likely be confined to bed still but at least we won't have to be here.

When we came here a couple days ago I would never have guessed all the trials and tribulations I would face to hold onto you just a little longer. Not only have I been heavily medicated but, also, nearly poisoned by magnesium sulfate. I am unable to move from my bed and therefore have been catherized so that they can measure the output of my urine to make sure the magnesium is making its way through my system. I feel like a giant slug who can barely move forward, and referred to myself as such to a dear friend of mine today. She thought it was funny. I'm glad to provide joy to someone in my current state.

Today I was allowed to eat my first solid food in almost 24 hours. I thought I'd be an unstoppable force attacking plate after plate of food, but instead barely made it through some cereal and a biscuit. Your daddy helped me finish it off. Waste not want not. Now I'm restricted to a liquid diet. Yummy!

Speaking of your daddy, he has been a trooper through all of this. He hasn't complained to me once. He won't talk about his feelings, though I'm sure they are mixed and confusing. He has been wonderful. He even gave me a sponge bath, or the equivalent of one. I hope when you get here you are like him, because he is so much stronger and braver than me. I've been in tears and openly stressed; he's held everything together like some sort of epoxy! (Which is a joke clearly meant for him.) I couldn't have chosen a better man to stand by my side, nor a better father. I can't wait for him to meet you. That will be the best moment of my life.

So far the good news is that you are measuring about a week ahead of schedule and they were able to get through both rounds of steroids to help make sure your lungs are developed in case you make an early entrance. I hope you don't. I hope you stay where you are for ten more weeks. I don't care what they put me, or my body, through in order to get you there. I will take it all on for you.

One final thought for today, and then I will write you tomorrow (medicine affects pending), I hope when you read this you do not see it as me blaming you for anything. None of this is your fault. I've learn, in life, that sometimes unpleasant things happen that we can't change or help. We just have to remember, always, that someone, somewhere out there, has it so much worse than us and that we should constantly be thankful for what we have no matter how hard or small. Things may be hard for us right now but I tell you what my darling little Remi, I wouldn't do anything differently if it means you will be safe and healthy when you make your debut. I'd do it ten times over just for you. I love you Remi-Roo! And I know by all those kicks and rolls you love me too.

I'll talk to you soon little dove.

Love always,

Mommy

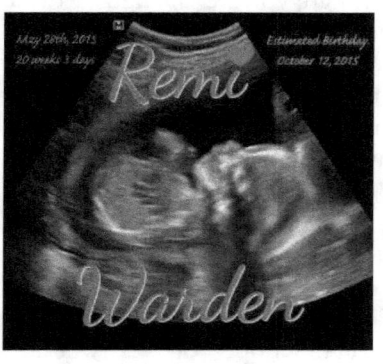

Still 29 Weeks 2 Days
July 29th, 2015

Dear Remi,

So, I know one day you will come up to me and request something of the most importance to you, and I will probably roll my eyes internally at how silly it all is. On the outside however, I will nod in encouragement and support because that's what I want to be for you. I want to be your rock that you bring all your problems to. I want to be your home you always willingly return to in your time of need. I want to be your safety. Because one day if you ever end up in a place like the one where I am at now and have to deal with the ups and downs of all of this I want to be by your side laughing with you at the results of a latex sensitivity in regards to a catheter, and a belly full of gas.

I love you little dove. Now to fall asleep to the sound of your precious heartbeat.

Love always,

Mommy

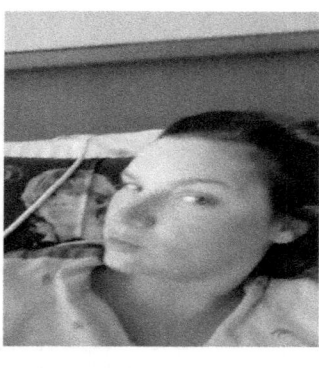

29 weeks 3 days
July 30, 2015

Dear Remi,

My hands are shaking so bad I can barely write this to you. Even autocorrect is confused by my words. The doctor came in to check my progress. We are thinning out…which could mean the worse. They stopped the magnesium and FINALLY took out the damn catheter. Sorry bad language already, but I am relieved! They gave me more shots of a medicine I had before to maybe help us. We also get two other medicines soon. I feel like my body has been taken over by the medicine. I'm shaking so bad I can barely focus. I hope you can't tell. I hope you are snug and warm and unbothered by all of this. I hope it all works for you and you get to stay like that a little longer. I hope you get to stay safe. Stay safe little Remi.

I love you.

Love always,

Mommy

Still 29 weeks 3 days
July 30, 2015

Dear Remi,

I've learned some things this morning while attempting to pee in a bedpan (which literally meant using my own bladder on its own for the first time in three days):

1) Nurses are wonderful people who are underpaid (I am sure).

I've done my best to refrain from being too emotional in front of the ladies here. I know this is their job and I feel that becoming an emotional burden on them does not make their lives better. However, after trying to lift myself up off a bed with muscles I haven't used in so long and agreeing to sit on a plastic pan to relieve myself I have come to realize how special these ladies are. They show so much compassion when they do not have to. They have helped me survive these last few days more than anyone else. I wish I could thank them appropriately.

2) When you need to cry, just cry.

I don't care who sees you – you should just let it out when you feel the need. Crying makes things feel so much easier to bare. It opens up a hole in your soul so all the negative can flow out. Do it and do it as often as you need to.

3) Peeing in a bedpan really isn't all that bad.

It is strange the first time around but it feels amazing to actually pee on your own. Speaking of which I need to do that now. Guess the next thing to get use to is having someone around to help you go! I feel like a baby again.

Love you little dove. I'll talk to you soon.

Love always,

Mommy

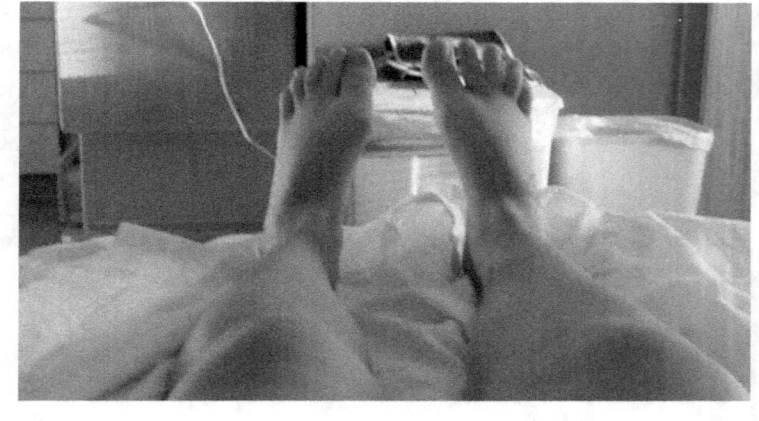

29 weeks 3 days still
July 30, 2015

Dear Remi,

My toes are like swollen pink sausages. I doubt I could fit into my shoes. My entire bottom half has transformed into almost a swollen waterlogged fish. I feel like I have tiny pillows all around my joints which makes it hard to judge distances. According to your dad I'm like a version of a little Asian grandma. I think that's kinder than bloated waterlogged fish but I call things as they are most of the times.

If you can't tell, I am feeling 100% better. I'm still tethered to my bed but with daddy's help I can maneuver to the toilet if I need to. I honestly forgot how good it is to pee in a toilet. That may seem weird but I'm telling you, it feels so good! I just finished eating some hospital food and literally thought I was gonna poop my (mesh underwear) pants before your daddy could help untangle and unplug me so I could get to the toilet. And of course as soon as I sat down I just peed. Don't shame the pee, it felt wonderful. It was just fun watching your daddy go go go as soon as I said what I needed. He's hilarious! Also, very helpful. As a side note: if I never have to have my blood pressure taken again in my life I think I'll be a happy person. There's only so much arm pinching one can take! Love you little dove. I will write again soon. Keep on growing in there.

Love always,

Mommy

29 weeks 4 days
July 31, 2015

Dear Remi,

I barely slept last night; the hospital bed isn't the most loving on your back, so excuse me while I wake up a little more.

We left the hospital today. We are in the car with your daddy and what remains of Dunkin Donuts, on our way home FINALLY! I'm so relieved to finally be out of there. I can't wait to be in my own bed again. But on the flip side I'm terrified of what could happen. I'm terrified this might cause you to come early. So stay in there a while longer little one. And in the words of your daddy stop overacting uterus and stay strong cervix!!!

I love you.

Love always,
Mommy

Still 29 weeks 4 days
Still July 31, 2015

Dear Remi,

Sitting at home now I honestly don't know what to do with myself. I can barely control my body, and standing up alone takes time.... everything is just so exhausting. I've settled into a depressed state I don't know how to recover from.

As a side note, our insurance may not cover the medicine I need to keep my body from continuing preterm labor. Your dad is trying to sort it out now, and hopefully they can. I really don't want another hospital stay under my belt.

I'm feeling horrible, Remi. I feel like I have just experienced the most traumatic week of my life.... like I was honestly tortured....and I don't even know if it is going to work. We don't know if anything is going to work. We know nothing and that's the part that bothers me the most. I'd like to say that I am okay because you are okay.... but I'm not. I have this deep down feeling that our relationship is being jeopardized because of this tragic week. I feel almost resentful even though I'm trying so hard not to. I know when I finally meet you this will all pass away from my mind. Until then, however, I'm unsure as to how I'm supposed to move on. No one will ever understand the emotional toll this has all taken...I'm not sure I even do right now.

I guess only time will tell.

Your soon to be very apologetic,

Mommy

29 weeks 5 days
August 1, 2015

Dear Remi,

Today has been better than the last week. Honestly though it is starting to hit me how much time we have left to wait on you. We have forever! Or it feels that way…. I had your dad pack our hospital bags in case you make your debut earlier than we'd like. We don't have many preemie clothes but we have a few just in case.

I've been having random contractions, some of which I think come from how I have been lying and where you kick me at. Also, I am feeling kind of down because the medicine I am on prevents me from feeling you move as much as normal. Any movement makes me happy to know you are okay even if I feel loopy.

I hope one day you look back on this and understand what it was like for us….and not just me but your dad too. He is being so helpful. I'm so blessed to have such an awesome man in my life.

We are blessed.

As a side note: I think I have lost 8 pounds in one day just from peeing off all the water weight I have gained. I'm slightly disappointed that I have to miss work next week (and for many more to come). I have so much I need to do to set up for the new school year that now I can't.

It is hard to know I have to give control of my work life to someone else. I'm not good with giving up control of anything, which is probably why this bed rest thing is so hard for me. I am a go go go do do do kind of person, and bed rest doesn't allow me to do either.

It is frustrating but at this point I'm really just

waiting impatiently for our next doctor's appointment to see how we are holding up. One day and one week at a time. We will get there…. even if I go crazy in the process.

Love always,

Loopy Mommy

3: 30 WEEKS

Dear Remi,

I have nearly made it through another day and you are now 30 weeks which is awesome! Today has been slightly easier. I can move around a whole lot better though I am not really allowed to, nor will your dad let me. The medicine still makes me very loopy but I am handling it better than before. I have barely had any contractions today at all. We don't have a doctor's appointment until Thursday and I have faith that we will make it until then.

It is super-hot in this house! I am sweating in places I shouldn't be! Also, I really really want a glass of chocolate milk but your dad won't go to the store and buy us milk and I can't go. Oh the dilemma of not being able to do things for yourself! Also, I did some work for my job today. It makes me feel slightly better about not being able to actually go to work. I know the amount of money we will be losing is eating at your dad. It is hard to stay on top of things when bad things keep happening. I mean first I had outstanding hospital bills to pay, and then $500 tuition to cover for class, then new tires, and now this…it seems like every time we turn around we have something else burying us under. Maybe one day we will be able to dig ourselves out of this hole. Maybe one day we will look back at all this hardship and it will just be a memory of what has made us stronger and better. I think if I can get through this year I can get through anything. Back to my "Malcolm in the Middle" Netflix marathon…I know I'm lame, but I have to have something to do!

I love you!! Stay in there and safe from all the horrible television while you can!!

Love always,

Mommy

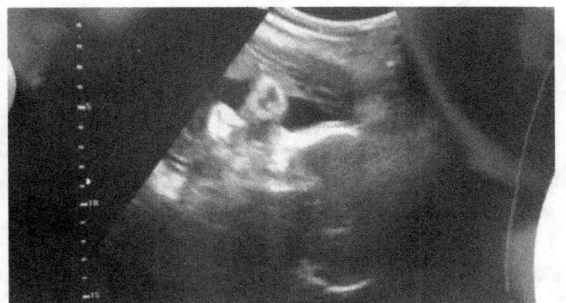

30 weeks 4 days
August 7, 2015

Dear Remi,

We had a doctor's appointment today. My blood pressure is fine, I've lost three pounds (probably from the hospital stay), and you heart rate was higher than it was before. It was 146; it was 130 something before that. I hope that's not the medicine affecting you. Other than that they checked my cervical length and it is fine, which is excellent news. Still on bed rest until I have you. The doctor actually said it took so much to stop the contractions it scared him. He really thought you'd be here by now, and he doesn't want me doing anything. I have a work note that says I cannot work for further notice.

The ultrasound tech tried to get a profile picture but your hands were in your face. They were like that for your 20-week anatomy scan too. Plus, you definitely were sucking your thumb. I hope you're not too shy, but being a little shy is okay. I enjoyed seeing you and knowing you are safe still. We go back to the doctor next Friday, where they will test us again to see if we might go into labor within the next two weeks and if my cervical length has changed at all. I'm excited to meet you but hope you stay at least another six and a half weeks so you can be 37 weeks and healthy….and so you for sure get to come home with us.

Ugh, I'm having a contraction right now and it sucks. I've had a couple random ones over the past few hours and they tend to make my back hurt pretty bad. They kind of feel like an ace bandage is being wrapped around my middle and pulled tight. I hope they stop. I don't want to go to the hospital again. I don't want you to be this early.

Your fur brother keeps knocking my hand for attention. His name is Calcifer and I can't wait for you two to meet. Also, I received my whooping cough vaccine today and so did your daddy. He was kind of surprised when they gave it to him, like it is just a women's doctor. However, it turns out they opened a family practice too. We, also, get to meet your potential first doctor next week.

We spent some time at our friends' house this afternoon. I don't know if not being home made me start having contractions again or what but they are bad tonight. It could, also, be that I haven't pooped really well in a while and could be constipated. I'm sure it doesn't help. Now your fur sister, Kayco, is nuzzling me for attention. I guess they missed us today.

I've come to better terms with having to be on bed rest for your health and safety. I feel better about it, though it is still hard. Two people I know delivered healthy full term babies today and that makes me sort of sad. I want you to be a healthy full term baby.

I know all these thoughts are random but that is kind of how my brain works nowadays. It is hard to focus on one thing, or remember anything, with all the thoughts and worry floating around in there. Hopefully it gets better. One day at a time is how I am dealing.

I love you.

Love always,

Mommy

4: 31 WEEKS

31 weeks
August 10, 2015

Remi,

We have made it through yet another week little Remi. Yay!!! I'm glad you are holding out. All these things happening around you has me on edge about how I'm even going to handle being a mother. I know I can take care of someone else; I've done that before. I, also, am not too worried about money. I'm worried about my emotional state going into this. I'm supposed to be strong and fierce. I'm supposed to be able to handle not just cope with things. I'm trying not to stress out...I'm trying to be okay. It is hard to be okay with everything I can't control. One day you will see just how in control of things I need to be. In other news, your dad's car is still messed up and I still don't know what's going on in regards to my work. I don't know what paper to file with who or who needs what from me. I'm stuck just waiting on that too. I guess this is what happens when you ask God to give you patience. I love you.

Love always,
Mommy

31 weeks 3 days
August 13, 2015

Dear Remi,

Last night your father and I watched part of the Perseid meteor shower. We didn't see very many, but we weren't out watching for too long. Looking at the sky like that; watching for lights randomly shooting across the sky, is exciting and scary. We are so small Remi; smaller than we accept most of the time. The universe is huge and we are tiny specks of dust compared to it. It makes everything I am dealing with seem meaningless and unimportant. Looking at the big pictures puts so much in perspective. It makes me feel better about surviving all that's ahead of us.

But then, it makes me think that this is the world you are coming into. Is this world really where I want you to grow up? This place is scary. There are terrible things all over the news every day: murder, rape, burglary, shootings, etc. I know much of what is reported is almost like scare tactics or because it sells newspapers. But the fact that it happens at all scares me as your mom. I just want what's best for you, which is why I'm lying here right now. Today I'm watching Daredevil on Netflix and eating cinnamon rolls, so perhaps not all things are bad in this world.

I love you.

Love always,

Mommy

31 weeks 6 days
August 16, 2015

Dear Remi,

We went to the doctor on Friday and there was still no change. We saw a new doctor who had no idea what has been going on and was talking to me about walking around to help the pain I am having in my back. Can't really walk around on bed rest can I? I wish they could just tell all the midwives at one time so I don't have to keep telling them. It frustrates me how horrible their customer service is there.

We stopped by Megan and Derrick's for a little while afterwards. It was just like being at home because all I could do was sit on the couch. There was good food and I'm sure that made your Dad happy since he didn't have to cook it. They bought us materials to make you more cloth diapers. It was the first time I ever made one and so that was an adventure. It turned out okay so I made three more. I really hope this cloth diaper thing works out because if not I'm going to feel really crappy.

I still can't get used to not being able to do anything. I hate it so much. I can't wait until we hit 37 weeks and we are safe. I want to walk around outside and clean the house and cook!! It is crazy how bad I want to clean!

Also, when we were at the doctor's they did an ultrasound and we finally got to see your face!! You have chubby cheeks just like me. I'm so excited to see you. I'm getting more and more nervous about giving birth to you naturally. If we make it to 37 weeks, I still plan on doing a water birth. If I don't then I'm probably going to get an epidural. Mostly it sucks being strapped to a bed in the hospital and I don't think I could handle the pain without moving around...and if you come early I doubt they will let me move around very much. We will see how things go.

I have classes that start next week. I am wondering how they are going to go with everything else going on right now. I finally had a substitute assigned while I am off work. However, he may want me to write lesson plans for him instead of him doing his own. That, plus classes, plus you.... I just don't know this is going to work out. I will figure it out though. I will. I am determined.

I love you.

Love always,

Mommy

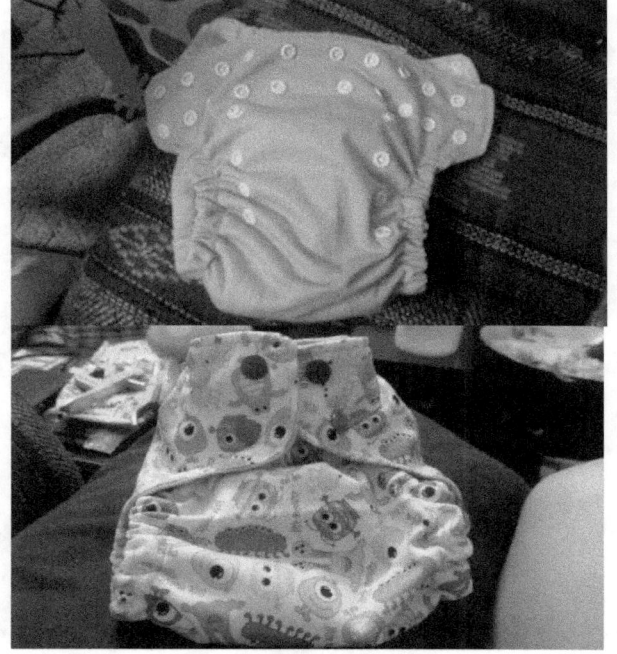

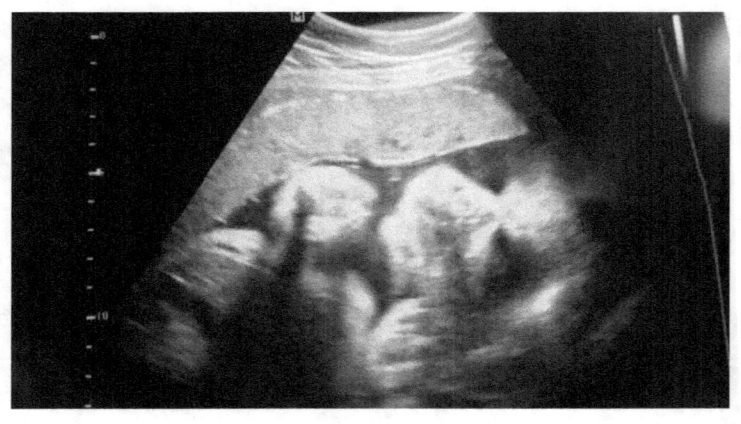

5: 32 WEEKS

32 weeks 1 day
August 18, 2015

Dear Remi,

Look! We made it to 32 weeks. That was our first milestone the doctor wanted us to meet and we made it! Congrats little girl.

I haven't finished making your diapers because I ran out of snaps. Your dad said we would get more later so alas my project has stalled! In other news, I have classes that start next week. I'm not sure I should be taking classes with everything going on, but life must continue.

I was approved for twenty days of sick leave from work. That's good, but I have to reapply to get more and they may not approve it this time around.

I repacked the hospital bag today. I still don't have everything together that we need but I don't know where we are going to end up having you so it is hard to know what to pack.

I'm starting to get really nervous about having

you. I don't know if I am brave enough or strong enough to have you naturally. If I end up having you in the hospital I'm about 100% sure I couldn't have you naturally, not with all the monitors and stuff attached to me. I want to have you naturally though. I want you to come into this world without drugs going through your veins. I want you to have the best start. I can't wait to have you here with me, but have no clue how I am going to handle work, school work, house work, and you. I'm lucky to have your father and his family. I'm luckier than I realize.

I started having diarrhea today. I worry that it is a bad sign, that I am going to go into labor soon. I was hoping to make it to at least 34 weeks without any more issues. I would love to make it to 37 weeks but I don't know how likely that it. I guess we will have to wait and see. Patience is one thing I lack, and the one thing you are teaching me.

I love you.

Love always,

Mommy

32 weeks 2 days
August 19, 2015

Dear Remi,

Yesterday afternoon and last night were rough. I was having contractions that should have sent me to the hospital. However, they finally slowed down so I didn't go in. I had your dad go to the store and get some Epsom salt for me to bathe in. I don't know if that helped or my eventual going to sleep.

Today they have come back a bit but they are irregular. That's a good thing I guess. I go to the doctor in two days so they will check me then and see if we are still okay. I hope we are. I thought we were doing so well and now all this...

My substitute from work came to see me today and talk to me about classes and lesson plans. He won't be writing lessons for me; he is too new of a teacher and doesn't feel comfortable doing it. It is okay. I'll just be set for the rest of the year.

I don't know how to deal with all this sometimes...but I am...and I will. I love you.

Love always,

Mommy

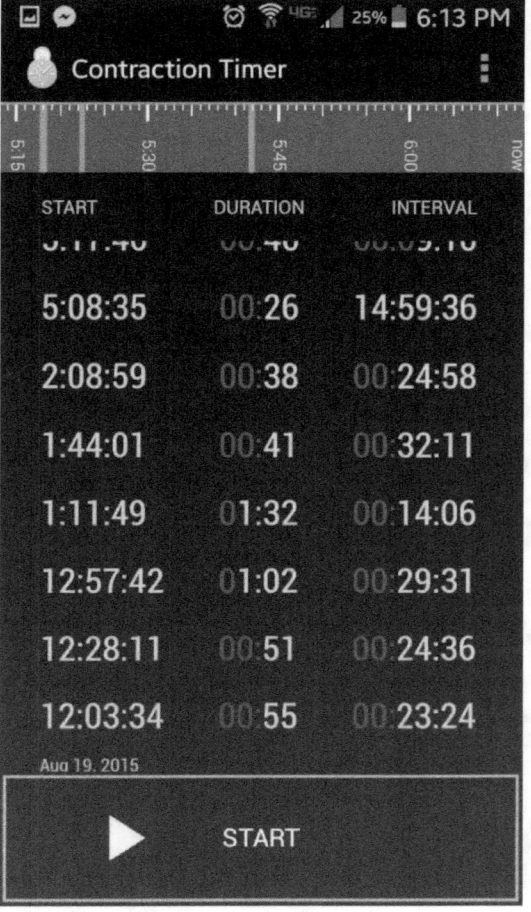

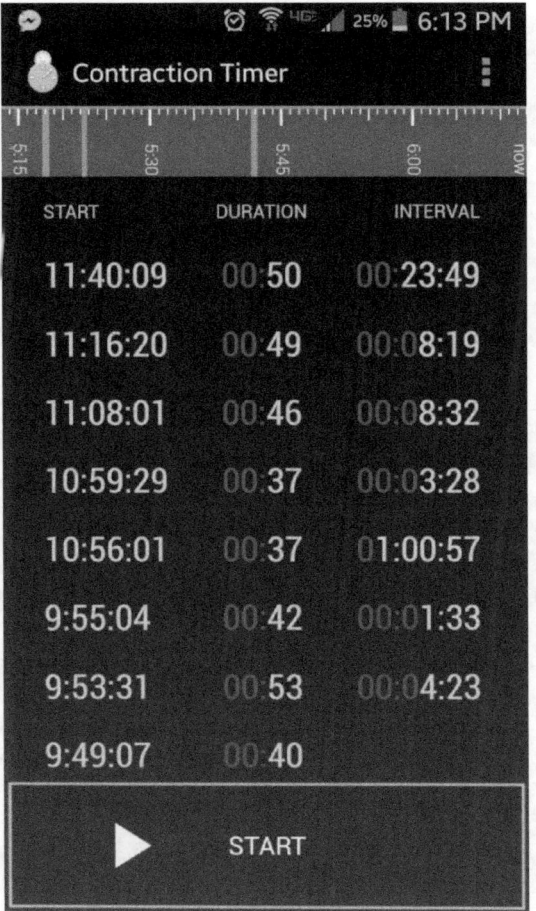

32 weeks 6 days
August 23, 2015

Remi,

Your grandparents and aunt came to visit us today. Your grandfather's uncle passed away and they have to his funeral to go to today. So many people are dying around us. A lady I work with gave birth to her twins a couple weeks ago. Her little boy had some issues and passed away. Her little girl is doing well, but I just can't help but feel absolutely awful for her. This isn't the first time that has happened to her; she lost a little boy before. I just keep thinking what if it was you? I wouldn't be able to go on with my life. We are getting closer to being far enough along that you should come home healthy and happy...or have a minimal stay in the hospital. I just hope you wait.

I made you some more diapers, because obviously I do not have very much to do with me time. Also, the classes I am taking start tomorrow so soon I'll have that to deal with.

Our doctor's appointment went well on Friday. I didn't have to have my cervix measured because apparently they stop doing that at 32 weeks. They said I'll be off bed rest at 36 weeks but I want to make it to 37 so I can have you at the birthing center and not the hospital.

The doctor gave us conflicting information about the medicine I am on. She said it doesn't actually stop contractions just stops me from feeling them. I looked it up and it says it blocks calcium to smooth muscles like the uterus which needs calcium in order to have contractions. I don't know which one is true, or if they both are and I just don't understand it. I wish doctors would explain things where we can understand them and don't make us feel like absolute idiots because we don't get it.

Work still hasn't figured out the sick days thing, so we may have no money for a while until the disability kicks in. I hate getting disability but we have to pay bills and eat.

I'm sorry every letter is stressful and not loving. I'm sorry that you will be entering this world with everything all topsy turvy. And here I thought you probably inheriting my cellulite and endometriosis would make your life hard enough. I guess that's what I get for wishing you the best.

I love you anyways.

Love always,

Mommy

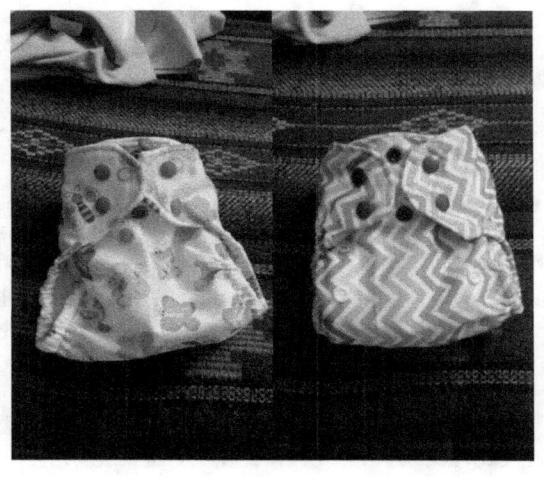

6: 33 WEEKS

33 weeks 3 days
August 27, 2015

Remi,

For the past few days I have been consumed with school work. The semester started on Monday and I already have so much to do...that and writing lesson plans for work. That's why I haven't written in a while.

It feels like autumn outside right now. The temperatures are wonderful! I just want to sit outside and eat pumpkin pie. I love pumpkin pie. Your dad actually made one for me, but now it is basically gone. It was really good. He's such a good guy.

I am waiting on paperwork from my doctor's office so I can try to get my short term disability – that way we can live! It had been rough not knowing how we are going to pay our bills. I wish the United States was like other countries that pay for maternity leave. I don't know why we don't have it when we pay so much in taxes as it is. I mean they take like one third of my paycheck for taxes and what do I get for it? Assistance?

Not even a penny. It is depressing.

On a sunnier note, you still are not here yet! I want to meet you but I am willing to wait. I am starting to feel kind of crappy, probably because I haven't been able to move around as much as I want. On the days when I do even a little bit too much I end up having contractions, so yay for doing nothing! We have to make it at least another 3.5 weeks to get to 36 weeks and then they are taking us off the medicine and bed rest. They want me to get to at least 38 weeks. That would be great.

Originally I wanted to have you naturally at the birthing center (where we see the doctor and midwives). I would actually be having a water birth. However, if you come early then we have to go to the hospital, where I will undoubtedly be strapped to a bed with an IV and monitors. With that in mind I think if we end up at the hospital that I am going to get an epidural, or maybe some other form of pain relief. If I get to use the birthing center, and the water and not being strapped down, I want to still have you naturally. Either way I have a plan, and I don't feel bad about taking the pain relief either. I thought I would, but I don't. I know what I can handle and what I can't.

I need to find a way to cheer up and not feel so yucky. Maybe sitting out in the sun would help a little, if only the bugs would go away! They see me as a yummy treat. It really annoys me. Daddy is making lunch now, while I watch television. I feel bad that I can't help him. I'll repay him one day.

I love you!

Love always,

Mommy

33 weeks 5 days
August 29, 2015

Remi,

I didn't sleep very well last night. Too many contractions, way too hot, and too much on my mind. I hate nights like that. I hate days like this. I'm sitting here in my bra and underwear burning up and feeling frustrated. I am so impatient with all of this. I want to be finished being pregnant but I don't want you to come too soon that you have issues or have to stay in the hospital. We don't have much longer to wait, and I know I can deal with it, but it is frustrating.

I'm watching Once Upon a Time right now. It is like a fairy tale soap opera. It makes the time pass by quicker though. I need to write lesson plans and do homework. I need to do a lot but I can't push myself to do it. I can't in case it causes issues.

Your dad cleaned the house a bit today, and now is at his ex-professor's house to help with a plumbing issue. I feel like we are not as close as we use to be. I mean we have so much strain on our relationship it is no wonder. I just hope things fix themselves sooner than later. I don't want to feel like I'm losing him too along with all this other stuff. I don't think I am. He's not mean or anything, more like stressed out and I can feel it. I don't know. I think the pregnancy hormones are getting to me. I love you.

Love always,

Mommy

7: 34 WEEKS

34 weeks 1 day
September 1, 2015 (2:40 am)

Dear Remi,

It has been a confusing couple of days dear. I'm currently lying in bed dealing with contractions. It is almost 3 am and I can't get comfortable and therefore I can't find sleep. I have an audiobook going called "Life as We Knew It." It is the first in a series which I'm listening to completely out of order, which is kind of how life feels like right now.

I feel like I should get up and eat something because I feel hungry, but then I'd have to find something, eat it, and then brush my teeth again. Oh man another contraction...ugh...

I am, also, dealing with a stabbing pain in my bladder (I assume it is my bladder). I'm going to ask to be tested for an infection when I see the doctor on Friday. My stomach had been super upset and gassy, and I feel like I need to poop constantly but I don't. All of this is so frustrating because I don't know what to worry about and what it just normal. Also, did I mention that I have to pee like every ten minutes? That has to be the worst part of all this. I'm jealous of your dad. He can fall asleep so easily and peacefully...unlike me.

I don't know if I should call the midwife about these contractions. I don't know what to consider normal and what should concern me.

You're moving around a whole lot right now. You keep stretching out and hindering my breathing, and jabbing me in the sides. It isn't too bad, though sometimes you hit a nerve. That's okay too...usually.

Another contraction... I'm waiting through them to see if they slow down. I can't wait to meet you no matter how terrified I am of labor right now.

I'm gonna go pee and try to sleep.

I love you.

Love always,

Mommy

Still 34 weeks 1 day
September 1, 2015

Dear Remi,

It is like almost noon! We survived last night!! I still feel uneasy and worry you will be coming any day now, but I'm starting to relax a bit today. Besides everything looks brighter and easier in the sunshine.

I love you.

Love always,

Mommy

34 weeks 2 days (technically) 12:11 am
September 2, 2015

Dear Remi,

So, guess what? We just returned from labor & delivery where we went after a day of fun fun fun contractions. They hooked me up to the monitors, checked me, and gave me two Brethine shots and sent me home. Better than the mag for sure!!! Dr. Casal showed up and said you looked like you were doing okay and that I should just keep doing what I'm doing. If the contractions return and are persistent then I'm to come back. Apparently I'm doomed to contract until I have you. I don't care, it is just good to be home! I just need to survive 3 more weeks and I'll be happy for you to come if you're ready. Three weeks, Remi!! Only three. It has been such a long long road I am getting nervous that we are so close. I'm nervous and excited and super SUPER thirsty!! I'm gonna go act like a fish.

I love you.

Love always,

Mommy

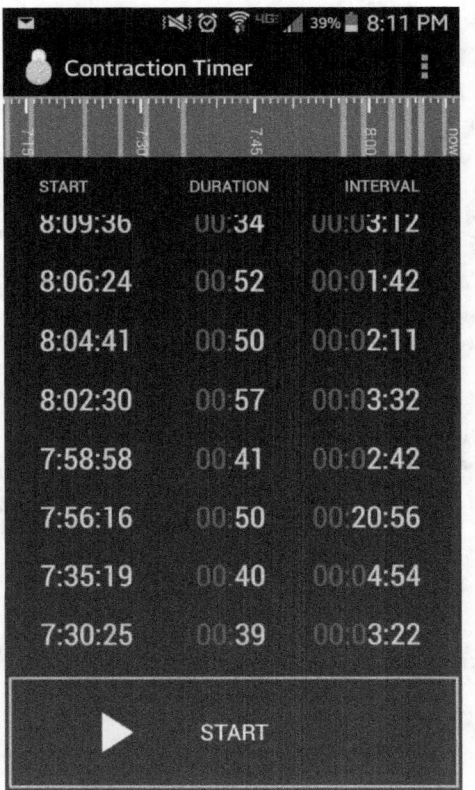

34 weeks 4 days
September 4, 2015

Dear Remi,

Today we had a doctor's appointment. Everything seems fine but I'm had contractions all day, even at the appointment. I feel like the doctors are not taking me seriously when I tell them how annoying the contractions are becoming. They have been happening for four days now...and they keep coming back. I do everything I am supposed to but to no avail. I think you just want to come out now.

I'm starting to feel weird about you being here. I wonder if that is normal? I bet it will change when I finally meet you...if hope so. In other news your dad is leaving me on my own for a night. I'm excited he gets to go have fun and I get some alone time. Also, I cut all my hair off...

You keep wiggling around but when I tell your dad to look you stop. Are you doing that on purpose?

I love you even if you are.

Love always,

Mommy

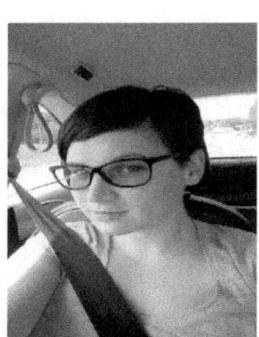

8: 35 WEEKS

35 weeks 1 day 11:23 PM
September 8, 2015

Dear Remi,

A lot has happened since we spoke last. To start off with the bad news first – your great grandfather on your dad's side (your grandfather's dad) passed away on Thursday (today is Tuesday). They had the layout on Sunday, which I didn't attend, and the service on Monday, which I did. I feel so awful for everyone in the family. I only met him a handful of times and he was already so different from how he was when he was younger, apparently. It makes me appreciate my new family so much more to see all the love they share. I feel bad for your grandfather...losing your dad isn't something I wish on anyone. It sucks so bad. I lost my dad when I was five, but I'm sure one day I'll share that story with you.

Anyways, the service was nice (if funerals can be nice). Your grandparents and aunt hung out with us afterwards, which is always fun.

I still haven't gotten my disability figured out. They are supposed to have the paperwork finished tomorrow but we will see.

I finished the lesson plans I needed to give my substitute before you get here which helps me feel a bit better. I still have so much homework to do though!!! I hope you are a baby that gives me the time I need to do it.

My (2nd) cousin had her baby on Monday; one day before she was to be induced. He is so cute!! He was 39 weeks and something and only weighed like five pounds. Such a tiny guy! I think you may be bigger than him already.

I've been having an awful week contraction wise. I feel so strongly like you are gonna make your appearance this week though I want you to wait until 38 weeks. I actually feel like you will be coming tonight, which is odd. I've been having contractions, lightning crotch (as it is called), back pain, and diarrhea (woot!). I, also, have another cold sore, which sucks!!! I know they are not for sure signs, but I have felt like today is the day since yesterday. I really can't tell you why. I even woke up stupid early this morning and cleaned some (oops!). I don't think it is full blown nesting but I am just so worried that this week is THE WEEK.

While we are on that subject, if you do decide to come this week, please excuse my frustration. I mean I had a plan little lady and you are ruining that plan! I wanted a natural water birth in a calm place that wasn't a hospital, but nooooo you just had to come early. And, if you don't come early, I would like to say thank you for allowing me to go through probably one of the most painful times of my life for you. Either way I love you. :)

Also, daddy and my friend, Stephen came to visit us today. It was nice to see him we haven't seen him in so long. We haven't seen anyone in so long. You will get to meet him soon enough I'm sure. I will talk to you soon. I love you.

Love always,

Mommy

P.S. Thanks for the kicks in the side and the ribs. They are oh so comforting!!

35 weeks 3 days
September 10, 2015

Remi,

So today I haven't had any contractions which is freaking me out probably more than it should. I am half tempted to call the midwife and tell her, but fear my freaking out about not having contractions may make her question my sanity.

In other news, I think I lost part of my mucus plug just now. It wasn't a lot so assume it is coming out in pieces.

Also, I got my paperwork back today and emailed it to the people who need it. I hope they take care of it soon. We need money. It is only because of family generosity that we have survived this long.

I have so much homework to do and have slacked so much this week. I guess that's what I'll be doing tomorrow. We are supposed to have people over on Saturday to hang out. It makes me wonder if you plan on coming tonight and so we won't actually have anyone over. It seems like something you would do...you sneaking little girl. I hope you hold off for your sake and because I have two cold sores and will be unable to kiss you if you come now. I don't know if me having them will make you sick either, so hold on a little longer.

Yesterday your dad and I got into a fight. We haven't had a fight in so long it made me super upset. It was all over me trying to finish your mobile before you get here and him getting annoyed because I kept getting upset at it while having contractions. It was a stupid fight that was due to us being on edge from everything.

Side note: Today we went to Smoothie King and I had a pumpkin spice smoothie that tastes just like pumpkin pie. It was amazing!!!! Also, we went and looked at a statue your dad helped his professor make. It was interesting to see it in place.

Also, our Xbox 360 acted like it was going to poop out earlier. It just shut off without any reason. We assumed that it overheated so we unplugged it and it is working. This is important because I NEED that Xbox. My life would suck right now without it.

Your dad and I are watching a weird movie about people taking pictures that show the future. Weird but interesting. I love you.

Love always,

Mommy

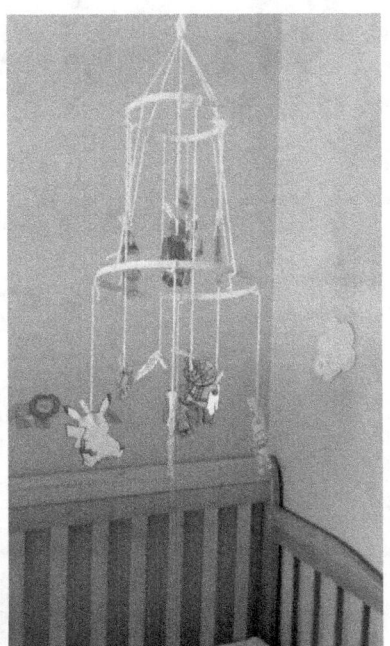

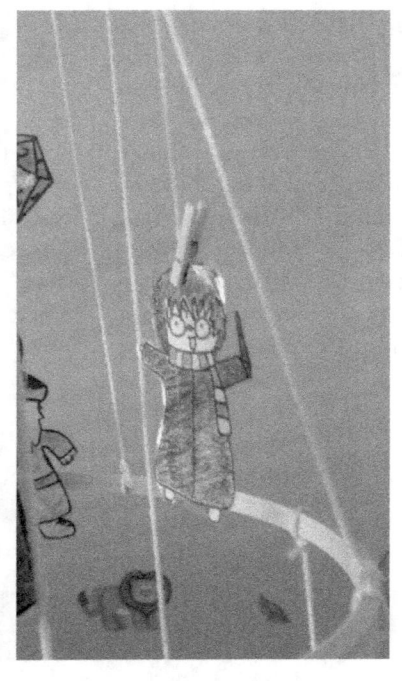

35 weeks 6 days
September 13, 2015

Remi,

Today is a lazy day (then again isn't every day). Your dad and I are watching TV snuggled up in the living room. It is kind of chilly outside and it feels awesome!!!

Yesterday some of our friends came over and spent the night with us. It was nice to have company. I did spend part of the day freaking out because you weren't moving as much as usually. I ended up drinking some knock off mountain dew to try and get you to wiggle some more. It didn't work, but eating dinner did. We grilled out chicken, pineapple, and onion kabobs, potatoes, and corn all made on the grill. It was yummy but I feel like I am paying for it today. My stomach is so gassy and I feel the need to poo, but can't. I have even been taking stool softeners to no avail. When I finally go it is going to be a madhouse!

So, tomorrow we are 36 weeks. That means we are off our medicine and if I have contractions again that they won't stop them at the hospital. We are on our own dear. It is going to be one long week! However, if we make it I can have you at the birthing center. I am excited to see when you decide to show up. I can't wait to see what color your hair and eyes are and to count your tiny fingers or toes!!! I'm nervous for labor but excited to have you out here with us. Hold on one more week little lady. I love you.

Love always,

Mommy

9: 36 WEEKS

36 weeks (!!!!!!!!!!!!!!)
September 14, 2015

Remi,

Today we are 36 weeks!!! Today we also take our last dose of Procardia. It is scary to think about what will happen without it.

No matter what I am ready for you. If we have to go to the hospital or get to have you at the birthing center, we have everything packed.

I really hope you hold on one more week and come next week. I have so many other things I want to do before you come and I want to give you the birth I feel you deserve.

I am starting to freak out on an epic scale. I know giving birth is supposed to hurt horribly but I know I have to do it for you. I just want things to go smoothly.

Last night I had trouble sleeping as well as a couple contractions, but nothing too serious. I, also, had a dream I started bleeding and had to go to the hospital. Let's hope none of that happens until next

Monday. I will keep you posted on how things are going. One more week little girl!! I love you.

Love always,

Mommy

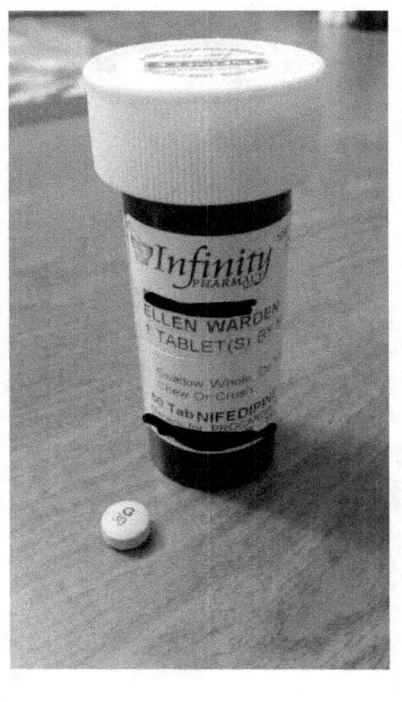

36 weeks 1 day
September 15, 2015

Dear Remi,

First day without medicine and we made it through! I'm so happy. It gives me hope that we will make it the rest of the week. I'm so excited for next week because you can come and everything can be perfect. I'm totally nervous but not as afraid as I thought I would be. I'm doing okay. I hope you are doing okay to. It drives me crazy to not know exactly how you are.

We went to town today and I checked out the Wizard of Oz series from the library. I've been reading them as light reading.

Also, my disability and sick days were submitted, which makes me happy. We may actually get money soon.

Also, your dad is selling his first art piece! I'm so proud of him because it is an art piece from his thesis show. I feel bad to think it but the money he gets will help us out a lot while we wait on my paycheck. I want him to buy himself something nice though. He deserves it.

I'm having occasional contractions but none too bad. Also, I feel like my mucus plug is slowing coming out (which is kind of gross). I know that it doesn't mean anything about a specific date but it tells me it won't be too long.

I really think it'll be next week. I guess we will see. I love you.

Love always,

Mommy

Facebook Post from 36 weeks
Posted 36 weeks 2 days, September 16, 2015

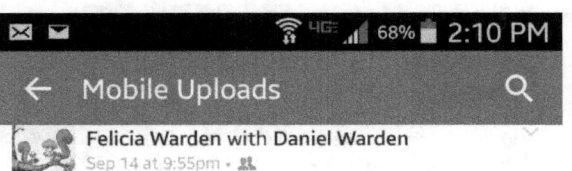

Felicia Warden with **Daniel Warden**
Sep 14 at 9:55pm ·

This picture is important and symbolic to me... At 29 weeks I went into preterm labor, which sent me to the hospital where I spent nearly a week, heavily medicated on magnesium sulfate, in order to prevent labor from continuing. It almost didn't work...the doctor was so sure I was going to have my baby. After days of vomiting, not eating, and feeling like death, I finally was able to go home, but with conditions. I had to take medication and stay off my feet on bed rest as much as possible. This meant I couldn't go to work, despite the new school year starting. It meant that my husband couldn't go to work all the time either in case I needed something or labor started again.

This picture is important because it is the last dose I am required to take now that I have hit 36 weeks. Over the last eight weeks I have been, not only taking this medication, but fighting for something important: my daughter's health and happiness. I have taken it twice a day, every day without fail. I have, also, been limiting my activity as much as possible, which meant not working, not helping around the house, not being able to get myself food, or do my own laundry, not being able to drive myself to the doctor, or go shopping. It meant depending solely on my husband to do pretty much everything for me, as well as support me through horrible contractions, self doubt, and fear. And yes,

 Write a comment...

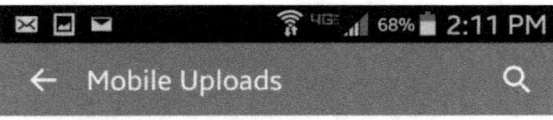

maybe you think that all of this is his job because he is my husband...and maybe part of that is right, but not fully. He didn't have to go buy me material for pointless crafts I decided to work on. He didn't have to buy me ice cream to cheer me up, or fill up my water bottle every time I asked. He could have told me to find something else to do in my free time, that I didn't need ice cream, or I could wait for more water. He never promised me these things, but he did them and is still doing them as we wait through this last week of my bed rest to end. He is amazing and one day I will pay him back, but until then I will keep this picture as a reminder...a reminder of what we went through together to get where we are now...a reminder of what we did together for our daughter. And though I may have taken my last dose, and though this may be my last week of bed rest, I know that no matter what happens we will continue to fight for each other and our daughter no matter what. We are stronger together and I know, no matter what, we will always be here for each other. No matter what our love will make us strong.

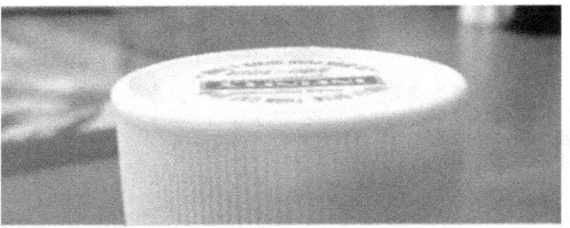

36 weeks 2 days
September 16, 2015

Remi,

I went to bed super early even though I woke up at like noon yesterday and then I woke up at noon today. I don't know what's wrong with me. I guess that I am just getting more and more exhausted.

Tomorrow I have a "baby tea" to go to at my work. They want to celebrate you! They are buying us a glider rocking chair and making it short and sweet so we can come back home and relax. I think it is nice but I don't know how to react to all the kindness. In my life people really haven't been all that kind. I have had a rough life and it has made it hard for me to accept gifts without someone expecting something in return. I wish I could get over it, but it is like ingrained in me.

In other news: I feel like I need to go poop so bad and can't! I don't want to force anything because I don't want hemorrhoids. I know it is all anything part of pregnancy but I just don't want to deal with it.

I've had a few contractions today. I am going to chug some water and see if things get better. I hope so. I feel so so off today, possibly because of the being so tired. I really don't know. I love you. I will write later.

Love always,

Mommy

36 weeks 2 days 11:00 pm
September 16, 2015

Remi,

I've taken an Epsom salt bath, sipped some wine, smelled some tea tree oil and not I am lying here while you hiccup away.

I have had a few contractions and ridiculous gas. I don't what it happening but if you plan to come tonight it would be nice to know. I have lots to do and it is late. It sucks being 36 weeks and not 37 yet, because I have to go to the hospital at the first sign of labor instead of waiting to see if it is actually labor. They won't stop it even if I go in, so I don't know why I have to go right away. Things just get so much easier next week.

I'm watching TV right now trying to ignore the contractions. I'm hoping they stop soon. Obviously you'll know one way or another, but I'll keep you updated.

I love you.

Love always,

Mommy

36 weeks 3 days
September 17, 2015

Dear Remi,

I'm in a lot of pain right now. I'm about to get in the tub to see if it will stop. I wanted to write you before I do.

I woke up at 6:30 this morning and couldn't go back to sleep until ten. I woke up finally around noon. So, it has been a short day.

Anyways, we had a "baby tea" at my work and they bought us a glider chair and some other small gifts. They, also, had us a cake and some punch. It was very nice.

I appreciate them more than they know, even without the gifts. Working with such wonderful people makes work nice to go to. I actually miss it somewhat.

I'm gonna go get in the tub right now. I really hurt. I hope this isn't it. I hope it is just a flare up.

I love you

Love always,

Mommy

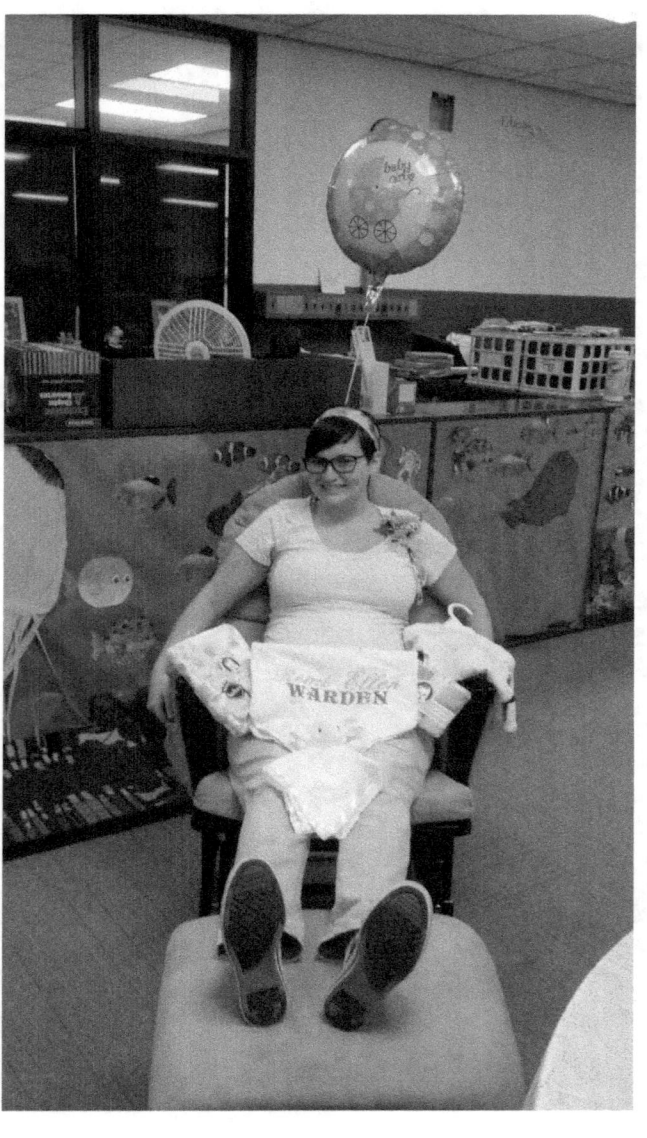

36 weeks 4 days
September 18, 2015

Remi,

I survived yesterday, thankfully. I barely slept though, due to horrible back pain. I think the weight of my belly is finally getting to me.

We had a doctor's appointment today. They did the group b strep test where they swab your vagina and butt. I should get the results Monday. They, also, measured my fundal (uterus) height and told me it is measuring 4 weeks behind. This made them have us go and get an ultrasound to see how you are doing. It turns out that you are still measuring ahead by about a week and your estimated weight is 6 pounds 15 ounces (nearly 7 pounds!). So, it is just your positioning that is causing the measurement issue. I have a little diaper rash like spot under my left butt cheek that I had them check out. I have had it for months and keep forgetting to ask about it. They gave me a prescription for some antifungal cream. They don't know what it is, but I'm ready for it to be gone.

We didn't get to schedule the birthing classes required to have you at the birthing center. She is supposed to call us about it Monday and let us know when. It is costing us an extra $65 to take the stupid classes, but we have to do it if we want to deliver there. I really hope my labor and delivery is everything I hoped it would be after all the hassle we have been through. I, also, hope I don't have you before the classes because then my plans are foiled again. I'm getting to the point where I just don't care when you come. I mean I want a specific thing but as long as you are good, who am I to complain one way or another?

We have our next doctor appointment next Friday. We have preregistration at the birthing center, a sizing ultrasound, and our regular appointment. I'm curious to see if the doctor is going to check me or not. He may just leave it be and let me go until you decide to come.

Oh gee I'm having contractions again...really annoying. I'm sitting in the tub trying to relax my back a bit. It seriously hurts.

Your dad had meeting today. He talked to one of the guys who originally stole the Tennessee Tech eagle that your dad has been working on copying. (That's a long story for another time.) It was a long meeting for me, but I filled the time looking for online birthing classes, because I am so worried about not taking them in time. Your dad told me I just need to chill. Well, it is hard to chill right now and I don't think he gets that!

I'm trying to get ahead on my homework right now, but have little motivation. I have so much work to do and I don't see how I am going to finish it. One of my teachers said I can finish my work by the end of next semester on an incomplete if I can't manage it. The other wants me to work ahead but there's only so much I can do at a time. I am going to try to finish all the work for that class this coming week to keep me preoccupied.

Oh, by the way, we are 37 weeks on Monday! That's really only a couple days away. I am so happy and proud that we have made it so far! I still can't believe you can come any time after that and be considered full term. I'm getting really excited. But let's not assume we will make it just yet. Anything could happen.

I'm gonna get out of the tub and try to relax now. The water is cooling off and not helping my back or the contractions. Remember it is just a little longer.

I love you.

Love always,

Mommy

36 weeks 5 days
September 19, 2015

Dear Remi,

Your dad upset me last night and so today hasn't been very fun. He got upset with me for saying that I didn't care how he cooked the food, because I was in a lot of cramping/contraction pain. It really bothered me because he yelled at me for saying I didn't care, without considering that I was too preoccupied to care. He, also, got all annoyed when I asked him to rub my back. I know I've been asking a lot of him and this hasn't been easy for either of us, but I think he just doesn't get that I don't have anyone else to help me. I should just let it go, but it hurts because my life has been so full of people getting upset with me for needing them.

It is hard to open up and let myself be vulnerable and so it hurt me more than it should. And maybe it isn't his fault, but he should understand…at least I think so. He knows my past. It hurts so much to feel like this. I just don't want any more help. I just want to do it all by myself and I can't and it hurts. It all hurts so much and it has all been so much it is overwhelming…

…and when you read this know that it is in no way your fault. I, also, know he never meant to hurt me like this. He was just having a bad day. But why does it hurt so much? Why does needing him and you hurt so much? Because believe it or not I love you and I need you already more than you know.

Love always,

Mommy

10: 37 WEEKS

37 weeks
September 21, 2015

Remi,

We made it! After 8 weeks of bed rest we are finally in the safety zone. I'm so proud of us.

I'm finally off bed rest too! We went to Nashville today to put money in the bank from where your dad sold that art piece. We finally paid the rest of our bills too. I bought a nursing bra at the mall and your dad bought a couple tools while we were out too. Bras are annoying and complicated trying to get the right fit. I hope the one I got works. Your dad, also, took me to Panera Bread to eat. I love their salads!!! We, also, went to Cookeville and ate at Shoney's with our friends Andrew and Aaron. Their food was terrible this time.

We finally have our birthing classes scheduled for Wednesday at 1 pm. I'll be glad when they are over with. I want to be completely set to have you, and that's the final thing we have to do. We have had a long long day and I am ready for bed. I walked around so much my whole body hurts! I love you. Stay safe, it won't be long now.

Love always,
Mommy

37 weeks 3 days (technically) 12:27 am
September 24, 2015

Remi,

We had our birthing classes today (well yesterday technically I guess). It cost us $120 to have the private classes which is frustrating while waiting on my disability to come in... She basically told us we are ready to do this. She was impressed with how much we already knew and said she wished all people came that prepared.

When we got home we repacked our hospital bags with some other stuff we needed. We are going shopping tomorrow (today) for some odds and ends for labor, like a light robe and some nursing shirts.

We, also, received some presents from your dad's aunts. We got a crib bumper set, changing table cover, and some other things. Everything is slowly falling into place for you. Our teacher said she thinks we will have a face labor but is worried that my overactive uterus might decide to quit halfway through which can stale labor. There are some tips she gave us for trying to make it progress if that does happen.

I think I over did it today. My back us hurting and your head is on my cervix very painfully right now. It makes it hard to get comfortable and sleep and I'm super exhausted! I don't know when labor is going to be but I think it should be Friday night. That is after our doctor's appointment and pre-registration, which would just be one less thing to worry about. I would be lying if I said I wasn't nervous because I am, but I feel confident I can do this – that we can do this. I'm gonna try and sleep. I love you.

Love always,
Mommy

37 weeks 6 days
September 26, 2015

Remi,

So, we had a doctor's appointment yesterday and we have not changed at all. It is sort of disappointing but okay. I think it is funny that we went from being upset by change to almost being upset by not changing. We still have like two weeks until your due date so it is okay. I'm not rushing you.

We are ready for labor though. We have repacked the bags and loaded them into the car. We still are waiting on your grandparents to bring us your car seat but they can do that the day you come for all it matters. It isn't like they live forever away.

We made some labor aide drink for me to have while I'm having you. It costs a bit of money to make but I hope it helps. It is supposed to help me not get so worn out. It has: honey, lemon juice, coconut water, water, rescue remedy, trace minerals, and sea salt. Consider it homemade Gatorade.

I, also, got sour suckers to help with feeling nauseous, a nightgown robe for laboring in, and a nursing shirt.

I think we are getting nervous and excited for you to get here. I just have to keep reminding myself that I can do this. I can have the birth we both need. But you never know what is going to happen...I love you.

Love always,

Mommy

11: 38 WEEKS

38 weeks 4 days
October 2, 2015

Remi,

So we made it to and passed 38 weeks. I haven't really felt motivated to write recently. I have been in some pain with you growing so big and putting pressure on so much. You keep kicking the same spot which is causing me a burning sensation. My back hurts and I can barely sleep because I just can't get comfortable. We registered at the hospital on Wednesday. Tuesday we went to Nashville with Daniel's ex-professor Bob. He needed a ride to the airport. Yesterday we worked on the eagle project your dad has to finish. We finally heard from the disability place and should get the check tomorrow. Hopefully, because we need to pay bills.

Your dad bought me an exercise ball to use as a birthing ball. He is getting everything I ask and doing everything I need. He just wants me to be comfortable during labor. We are ready for you, or as ready as we can be I guess. I keep having contractions but they are not doing anything.

Tomorrow we have some family reunion of your dad's to go to. We originally were not planning on going because of you…well if you showed up. Having a newborn seems to be tricky work.

We, also, got a flu shot today and went to the doctor. He felt around on you and said you feel small and are still head down. It is a waiting game from here on out.

I love you.

Love always,

Mommy

12: 39 WEEKS

39 weeks 4 days
October 9, 2015

Remi,

I woke up this morning, about 6:45, with what I assume was a bloody show and the loss of my mucus plug. I, also, had to poo but nothing too major. Maybe today is the day? I currently have some cramps but nothing specific and it is 7:11.

The past couple days I have had some pretty strong contractions. None were too painful. I feel like your head on my cervix is the most painful part so far. Right now I'm lying in bed next to your dad about to try to sleep some more. If this is it, then I need my rest for sure. It could just be the loss of my mucus plug and nothing else though. Only time will tell.

Your dad finally finished the eagle and took it off. I know he is so glad that thing is finished. He has other projects that he needs to finish but that's the one that was bothering him.

Multiple women have commented on how small my baby bump is considering how far along we are.

They keep saying I should be bigger or I don't look that pregnant. They told me that you have been measuring big though so I don't get that.

Oh man I'm definitely having contractions now. I called the midwife but no one answered. I don't know if I should call back or not...or just try to rest. Please don't pop out in the car, Remi. Even though that would be a story to tell.

I need to get up and eat and clean the house one more time since I won't feel like it later, but I think sleep may be more important. I think I'm gonna sleep then call them again when I wake up.

I love you.

Love always,

Mommy

13: BIRTH

Posted to Facebook
October 13, 2015 at 9:18pm

On Friday morning (around 6:30 am) I woke up with contractions and bloody show. I could not go back to sleep and am pretty sure between 630 and 9 my water broke (I had a high break but was unaware of this because it didn't leak continuously).

We called the midwife about being in possible labor and went in to see them at 1 pm. On the way there a young lady rear ended us, which is another story. We weren't progressed enough to stay at the birthing center so we went home to labor until around 11 PM when we called the midwife with stronger contractions and went in to be checked. We were 3 cm at the time of arrival and walked around the birthing center for an hour and were checked again and had progressed to 4 cm, so she admitted us. At the birthing center we labored naturally all throughout the night and day, being checked every four hours.

Our labored progressed up to 7 cms, but then I

stopped progressing. My midwife thought it might be because my water bag was partially intact and decided to rupture the rest of it to see if we would progress, but that caused her Remi's head to put too much pressure on my cervix which started to swell.

They waited four hours to see if it would change but the swelling put us back at 6 cm. Around 5 pm on Saturday they sent us to the hospital for pitocin and some pain medicine since we hadn't slept and they thought sleeping might calm things down.

The epidural didn't work even though they tried it twice but the pitocin did. It took us from 6 cms to 9 cms by 12 am. I had a slight fever and they talked about a possible c-section if it didn't go away. It thankfully did.

However, my cervix was still not fully dilated but they allowed us to start pushing to see if her head would cause change. She was delivered vaginally at 140 am. I had excessive bleeding and was given medicine to try and stop it.

We ended up having to stay an extra day in the hospital because my hemoglobin levels were low. They talked about a blood transfusion but luckily I recovered. Remi is slightly jaundice but did not require treatment for it. We are home now and doing well, just adjusting to our newborn schedule.

Overall I loved my experience at the birthing center and would love to have any future children there. I actually enjoyed my natural labor despite not being able to do the fully natural delivery. I had an awesome support person in Daniel and feel that we made an awesome team throughout everything. I know that we had to transfer for Remi's sake and feel happy with how things turned out.

14: POSTPARTUM

November 21, 2015
Almost 6 weeks postpartum

Remi,

Can you believe it? You'll be six weeks tomorrow!!! Wow so much has happened that I didn't write about, and that it will take me time to recall and relay. Right now you are sleeping beside me in your Dad and my bed because it is the only place you will sleep. It has been a rough six weeks. I hope when you get older and decide to have children of your own that I can openly tell you how hard this has all been. Don't worry though because you are truly worth all of it. I look at you sometimes and I am in awe. I love you more than I ever imagined I would or could. You are so extraordinarily special to me no matter how hard things have been. Plus, I know that things will get better. I am torn between you growing up a little so you can communicate with me better and you not growing up too fast so I can cherish this time with you. I will try to write again soon. I love you.

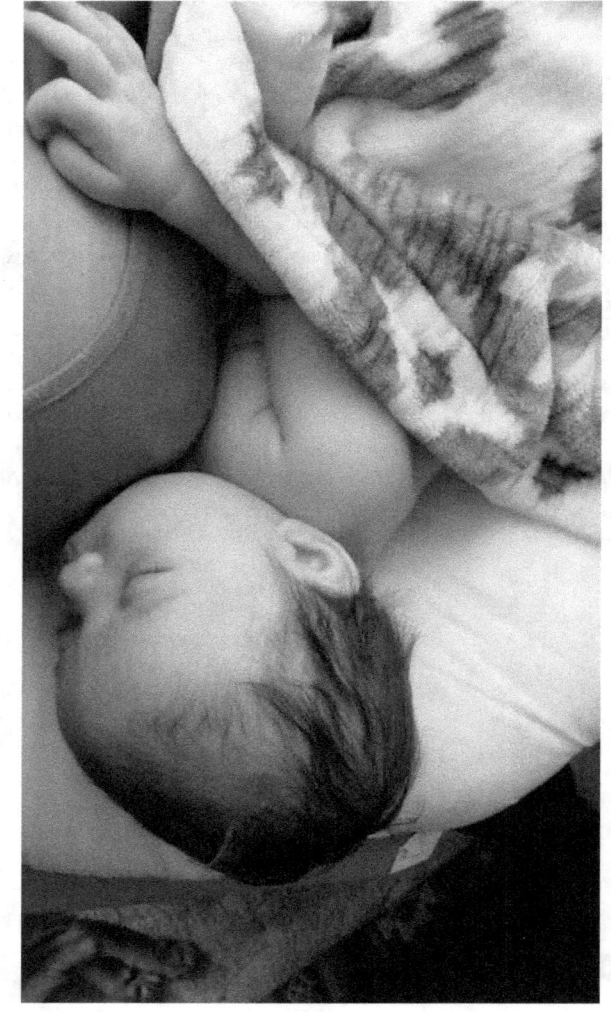

E. F. C. Warden

Love always,

Mommy

October 7, 2016
Almst One Year Old

Dear Remi,

This will be the last letter I write you on here. I wanted to end this with a letter for your first birthday.

The past year has simultaneously crawled and gone by too fast. You have become a very active little lady! You have been walking since you were 8 months old and stealing food from people since you were about 5 months, and those are just highlights of the past year!

You say momma, dada, chickey (chicken), tickle tickle (play), and you can sign milk, more, and all done. We think you think the sign for milk means momma, but that is okay with me. You throw a fit whenever someone is eating and doesn't share. You climb on everything you can get onto. You love love love splashing and playing in water - including the dog bowl. You like to try to eat acorns, rocks, and even dog food, when we go for walks. And you giggle and smile when someone tells you not to do something like we are cracking a joke. You hate having your diaper changed and love running around naked. You sleep with me and daddy at night and refuse to sleep alone and the truth is that I don't mind at all. It is actually nice.

You are the light of my life even though I will be the first to admit you are very very clingy and demanding. It is okay though. I enjoy our snuggles and playtime. I even enjoy being your comfort when you accidentally fall or are tired or frustrated - not that I want you to do these things but sometimes bad things are inevitable. I am just glad that I can be here for you. I will always be your biggest support no matter where life takes you. I will always love you unconditionally and without fail. There is nothing in this world that you could do to stop me from loving you. Even when you turn 14 and think the world is out to get you and that no one understands you or your life - I will be here loving you. Even if some days you "hate" me - I will be here loving you. You can talk to me about and tell me anything. I will always be your comfort as long as you allow me to be.

For your birthday I have decided to give you a wish as your present. I wish, for you, happiness, drive, and the unfaltering ability to chase your dreams and be yourself. I may be throwing you a party you will never remember but I hope you never forget my wish for you.

Remi, my dear, you are loved beyond words. Thank you for changing my life. Thank you for teaching me patience, acceptance, and what it means to love with all my heart.

Happy Birthday my sweet girl! I love you!!!

Love always,

Mommy

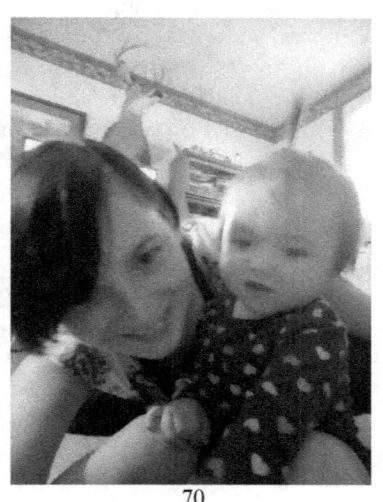

29 Weeks

ABOUT THE AUTHOR

E. F. C. Warden is the mother of one human and three animals. By day she works as a high school librarian, and by night is a mastermind multitasker while raising her daughter, writing, reading, and going on random adventures. She currently resides in Tennessee with her husband, daughter (who this book is about), dog, cat, and tortoise. This is her first book.